101 Tips for Parents of Kids with Diabetes

101 Tips for Parents of Kids with Diabetes

Wisdom for Families Living with Type 1

Jeff Hitchcock

Skyhorse Publishing

Skyhorse Publishing books may be purchased in bulk at special discounts for sales promotion, corporate gifts, fund-raising, or educational purposes. Special editions can also be created to specifications. For details, contact the Special Sales Department, Skyhorse Publishing, 307 West 36th Street, 11th Floor, New York, NY 10018 or info@skyhorsepublishing.com.

Skyhorse® and Skyhorse Publishing® are registered trademarks of Skyhorse Publishing, Inc.®, a Delaware corporation.

Visit our website at www.skyhorsepublishing.com.
10 9 8 7 6 5 4 3 2 1

Library of Congress Cataloging-in-Publication Data is available on file.

Cover design by Rain Saukas

Print ISBN: 978-1-63450-504-8
Ebook ISBN: 978-1-510-70582-1

Printed in the United States of America

To the Children with Diabetes Family

Table of Contents

Table of Contents

Table of Contents

Introduction

My family's journey with type 1 diabetes began in September 1989 when my daughter Marissa, then just two years old, was diagnosed. My wife Brenda and I felt confident in the words of her endocrinologist, who said, "We can make a big difference in her life." From Marissa's care team we learned how to check a finger-stick blood glucose, how to measure up her Regular and NPH insulins, and how to treat a low blood sugar. Brenda and I vowed not to let diabetes stop Marissa from doing anything she would have done otherwise.

Over the years, the tools we use to care for type 1 diabetes have changed dramatically. Finger-stick checking changed from two agonizing minutes to a few seconds. Continuous glucose monitoring (CGM) systems were invented and improved and now connect to cloud services. Insulin analogs replaced Regular and NPH. And insulin pumps became commonplace. But what hasn't really changed is what happens at diagnosis. Families are taught the same thing we were: the basic mechanics of caring for type 1 diabetes—the glucose monitoring, the carbohydrate counting, the insulin dosing.

But to be honest, those are the easy parts of diabetes care. The challenge is to learn how to fit diabetes care into your life, and then to get on with living—and living well. This book contains 101 bits of wisdom, collected by our family over the years, that were shared by others much wiser than I. Think of these tips as the footnotes on living with type 1 that your care team would share with you if they had the time. (And be sure to check out the Additional Resources section for websites, studies, blogs, and more mentioned in the tips.)

While the medical management of type 1 has changed and will change with advances in medicines and devices, I'm hopeful that the 101 tips within this book will be as meaningful years from now as they are today.

As you read this book, remember that I'm just a dad. Always work with your child's diabetes care team on any changes you might want to make.

Jeff Hitchcock
President and Founder, Children with Diabetes

1

Living Every Day with Type 1

Everyday life with type 1 diabetes requires a little additional thought and planning. These tips will help enhance your family life.

1 Life First, Diabetes Second

If our goal in caring for type 1 diabetes were perfect blood glucose readings, we could accomplish that—but doing so involves sitting in a hospital bed with an IV in each arm, every minute of every day, forever. So let's set that aside and assert that perfect blood glucose readings cannot be our goal, because to achieve that goal we'd have a life not worth living. Our goal has to be a life worth living, and thus diabetes care has to be second—an important second, but second nevertheless.

One of the first books my wife and I read about caring for our daughter was *Sweet Kids* by Betty Brackenridge and Richard Rubin. (Make a note: get that book.) In *Sweet Kids*, Betty and Richard, who would become good friends, turned on its head what was then the standard of care for kids with type 1 diabetes: they put life first and diabetes second. That philosophy of living your life and fitting diabetes into it has always been the driving goal for our family and for Children with Diabetes, the organization that I founded and run.

If you take nothing else away from this book, take that away—live your life as you always wanted, and figure out how to fit diabetes in.

2   It's Not Your Fault

After your child's diagnosis, you learned how to check blood glucose levels, determine carbohydrate contents in food, dose insulin, and treat low blood glucose levels. You overcame your fears and let your child return to school or play with friends. You also read a lot online about type 1 diabetes and what science knows about its underlying genetics and risk factors. You might be reflecting on the weeks and months leading up to your child's diagnosis, wondering what you did that might have caused it, or why you didn't catch it sooner. It's time to let those feelings go and to stop blaming yourself for anything. Based on the science of today, there is nothing you or anyone else could have done to prevent your child from developing type 1 diabetes. And unless you knew someone with type 1 diabetes, you probably wouldn't have thought your child's illness was anything other than a cold or the flu. So take this to heart: it's not your fault.

3   There Is No Cure—Yet

Let's get this out of the way now. Today, there is no cure for type 1 diabetes. No diet is going to change your child's life. There is no supplement that reverses type 1 diabetes.

Losing weight doesn't make type 1 diabetes go away. And you don't outgrow type 1 diabetes. There is only insulin, which your child needs every day for the rest of his life.

I mention this because you will come across claims of miracle cures, perhaps even by friends. Don't be fooled. Don't spend any money on them. And rest assured that the moment there is a cure, you will read about it on the front page of every newspaper, you'll hear about it on every major television news program, people will win Nobel Prizes, and your child's diabetes care team will celebrate with you and every other family living with type 1 diabetes.

4   Would You Allow Something without Diabetes?

As a parent, you're going to face many decisions about what to allow and not allow as your child grows up. There will be play dates, sleepovers, school sports events, class trips, vacations, even choices of desserts. When you add diabetes to the situation, you might be tempted to say no to a request because diabetes makes events and decisions more complicated. If you're getting ready to say no, I urge you to ask yourself, "If my child didn't have diabetes, would I say yes?" If you answer yes, then you have to find a way to make it happen with diabetes. You owe it to your child.

5   Learn in Stages

You don't need to become an expert in type 1 diabetes immediately to keep your child healthy. You do need to know a few things right away, including: how to measure blood glucose; what your child's target blood sugar range is; how to measure and inject insulin; how to treat a low blood sugar; and how to estimate insulin to cover meals. Those are the basic life support skills for type 1 diabetes. Day by day, you will get better at those skills, and you can then begin to learn more about type 1 diabetes and how to care for it.

Your diabetes care team is there to help you learn in stages. At diagnosis, and for the first days and weeks, they will help you as you master the basics. In later months, they will help you get better at estimating carbohydrates in food and teach you about insulin pumps and continuous sensing technology. They will also share with you the status of research into advanced care technology like the artificial pancreas and biological research into preventing and possibly curing type 1 diabetes.

My advice to newly diagnosed families is to take it slowly for the first couple of weeks, keep a list of questions for your diabetes care team, and don't be afraid to ask anything. Caring for type 1 diabetes is different for everyone. What works for one person might not work for you—or as my friend Bennet Dunlap says, "Your diabetes may vary."

6   Language Matters

How you speak about diabetes and diabetes care tasks really matters. First and foremost, use "check" instead of "test" for blood glucose monitoring. The word "test" has connotations of passing and failing, but you can never pass or fail a blood glucose check. You're just getting the data (more on that in a minute).

Another term that has no real place in diabetes care today is "compliance." You'll hear and read about "patient compliance" in medical journals and in some articles about diabetes. "Compliance" implies following someone blindly. That's not how we want to live. A better way to think about this concept is "adherence"—adhering to a care strategy that you and your care team have created that lets you and your family live the life you want while caring for your child's diabetes.

You'll also hear the term "diabetic," referring to someone who has diabetes, type 1 or type 2. There is great debate in the diabetes community about that term. We don't, after all, call someone with cancer a "canceric," do we? So my suggestion is that people who don't have diabetes should use "person with diabetes," and that people who have diabetes can use whatever term they like. You'll never go wrong saying "person with diabetes," but you are likely to upset a large number of people by saying "diabetic."

News reports often speak of someone "suffering" from diabetes. I loathe that term. "Suffer" implies a certain state of inability, pain, helplessness, and resignation to that situation. That is not what we want for our kids, and it is certainly never anything a parent should accept. We want our children to thrive with type 1, never suffer.

Finally, be mindful of the language you use when reacting to blood sugar readings that are outside of your child's target range. For example, if your child comes home from school and has a high blood sugar, don't ask, "What did you do? What did you eat? Did you forget to take insulin?" Instead, calmly say something like, "I see that your blood sugar is high. Let's talk about it and do what we need to do to bring it down."

7 Data Matters

The single most important bit of data we use to care for type 1 diabetes is the *blood sugar reading*. It doesn't matter if the reading is from a finger-stick blood glucose meter or a continuous glucose monitor. That data is what we use to determine the insulin dose, decide if it's safe to drive, determine if your child is prepared to take an important exam, and so on. And it makes sense that the more data we have, the better decisions we can make.

The single most important piece of advice I can offer is to get lots of *accurate* glucose readings. The second most important piece of advice I can offer, especially to teens, is never to lie about this data. (More on that later.) These readings are so important that each one should be cherished. It doesn't matter if the reading is low, in target, or high. It's data that you use to make a decision about care, and without good data, you can't make good decisions. Be grateful for every single reading.

8   Be Comfortable with Approximations

So, having said that it's important to get accurate blood glucose readings, I need to offer some qualifications. I often say that type 1 diabetes is an information-management challenge. That's because so much of the decision making in type 1 diabetes is about numbers: blood glucose readings, carbohydrate counts, units of insulin, duration of boluses (or intravenous injections). The real challenge is that the numbers that make up these data are not as precise as we might think. They are at best approximations and, as a result, a lot of what we do is not as exact as we'd like. To succeed mentally in diabetes, you must become comfortable with this imprecision.

A couple of examples will help make this clear. Let's start with blood glucose readings. All blood glucose meters—including the most accurate—have an error range of either a fixed number or a percentage. In the lower glucose range, the error is generally presented as a fixed number, such as plus or minus 20 mg/dl. In the higher glucose range, the number is generally presented as a percentage, such as plus or minus 20 percent. As you can imagine, there is quite a difference between 50 mg/dl and 70 mg/dl, as well as between 240 mg/dl and 280 mg/dl. Yet a "good" meter can vary that much in its reading and still be considered to be accurate.

Variability in carbohydrate counting can also be quite high. For packaged foods, sugar and carbohydrate values can vary by plus or minus 10 percent. For prepared foods, even the best-trained professionals are often wrong by as much as 20 to 30 percent in their estimates.

When you combine glucose reading errors with carbo-hydrate counting errors, it's easy to wonder how we ever get blood sugars in the target range. And those errors are often an explanation for why blood sugars one day don't match what happens on another day.

The important point is that you can do very well living with type 1 diabetes in spite of these approximations. And not expecting perfection can help reduce your stress levels.

9 When Sugar-Free Matters and When It Doesn't

You've no doubt seen an aisle in the grocery store with sugar-free products. Some might even be labeled DIABETIC. These foods include sugar-free pancake syrup, jellies and jams, and even candy. Many are sweetened with sugar alcohols. Sugar alcohols include sorbitol, xylitol, mannitol, lactitol, and others. While small amounts of foods with sugar alcohols are fine, eating too much can have a laxative effect, especially in children.

People with diabetes often buy these foods thinking that they have lower levels of sugar and carbohydrates and will thus not increase their blood sugar as much as the regular product. Given the laxative effect of sugar alcohols, my advice is to avoid sugar-free products as much as possible—especially the products that are sweetened with sugar alcohols. In our family, the only sugar-free products we used regularly were pancake syrup and soft drinks.

Another reason to avoid sugar-free foods is to learn to live in the real world. When your child is a teen and adult, out on his own, he will want to eat what his friends eat as much as possible. Teaching him to integrate regular food into his diet as a child will prepare him for success as he grows up.

10 What Your Child Can and Cannot Eat

Let's be very clear: Your child with type 1 diabetes can eat anything. Except poison. And cookies made from poison.

That bit of humor was created by a mom named Joanne Cunha in response to things people say to parents of kids with type 1 diabetes. (Check out her YouTube video and her blog. The links are listed in the Additional Resources section.)

But seriously, people with type 1 diabetes can eat anything, as long as you provide enough insulin to cover the carbohydrates in the food. As a parent, your job is to teach your child about healthy eating in general. Focus on that.

I'll add one caveat: any kind of liquid sugar is very hard to cover with insulin. That includes fruit juices, lemonade, Kool-Aid, and regular soft drinks. The sugars in these products will raise blood sugar extremely rapidly, and it's almost impossible to take enough insulin far enough ahead of consuming them to compensate for them. That's why we use them to treat low blood sugar.

11   Avoid "Diabetic" Meals

On the topic of what you can and cannot eat, I highly recommend avoiding "diabetic" meals at restaurants and on airplanes. These meals are generally designed for older adults with type 2 diabetes and may be high in fat to avoid being high in carbohydrates. When you're at a restaurant or traveling, eat what you would otherwise eat.

12   Thank Well-Meaning Friends and Relatives

We all have well-meaning friends and relatives who share with us the latest miracle cure or treatment that they've found online or heard about in the news. These are the same people who ask, "Will your child grow out of it?" and counsel against eating sweets when you're out to dinner. They are trying to help, but their help is usually not helpful. Thank them for their concern and let them know that there is no cure for type 1 diabetes, that type 1 is different from type 2, and that you and your diabetes care team work closely to ensure that your child can live a full life that includes foods that all of us eat. With that said, don't expect that you won't hear from them again when the next "miracle cure" finds its way into the daily news.

13   Find a Babysitter

Caring for a child with type 1 diabetes can be overwhelming. Be sure to make time for you and your spouse to go out alone, without your child. If your child is young, that means finding a babysitter you trust to care for a child with diabetes. Ask your diabetes care team, contact your local JDRF or American Diabetes Association (ADA) chapter, or check out the Safe Sittings website to find adults or teens with type 1 (or who have siblings with type 1) who live in your area and who can babysit for kids with type 1 diabetes. They already understand type 1 diabetes and will know when they need to reach you. If you have family close by and they want to help, you'll need to provide them with diabetes care training. If your child is older and can take care of herself for several hours, you should feel comfortable going out for the night. Cell phones, text messaging, and remote CGM monitoring all help. The important thing is to actually go out. You need an occasional break to keep your relationship healthy with your significant other.

14   Involve the Grandparents

Grandchildren need to know their grandparents, so be sure to teach them how to care for your child's diabetes. Some diabetes centers offer education sessions for grandparents. If yours does, take advantage of it. If it doesn't, teach your parents and your spouse's parents the basics, including checking blood sugars, treating low blood sugars, and injecting or bolusing insulin. With that knowledge, they'll be able to be actively involved in your child's life. That's very important.

15   Learn about National Support Organizations

When your child was diagnosed with type 1 diabetes, you no doubt asked your diabetes care team about national organizations that can help. You might have already known about the American Diabetes Association (ADA) and JDRF, the two largest and best-known diabetes-related nonprofits in the United States. ADA and JDRF do very different things, but both are important to families living with type 1 diabetes.

From the perspective of a parent, the ADA's most important programs are its focus on diabetes summer camps and its access to care at school. Diabetes summer camps (discussed later in more detail) offer kids with type 1 an opportunity to meet many other kids with diabetes, learn self-reliance, and build friendships that last a lifetime. ADA's Safe at School is a national program that works to ensure that kids with type 1 have access to appropriate diabetes care while at school and can participate in all school activities.

As a parent, you should learn about national and local ADA and JDRF resources that can help you, your child with type 1, and your family.

16   Find Local Support

While national organizations can be very helpful, local support can be even more so. Ask your diabetes care team about local support groups for families living with type 1 diabetes. Often parents of kids will form a group that meets occasionally to catch up on research news, share diabetes care strategies, offer each other support, and simply be together. In addition to offering support for parents, local support groups offer kids with type 1 and their siblings a chance to meet other kids facing the same issues they are. Even if the meetings are strictly social, they can be very important in giving you and your kids

14

a chance to share experiences that are unique to families living with type 1 diabetes.

17   Go to a Diabetes Conference

Imagine you walk into a room with over two thousand people, all families living with type 1 diabetes. You see toddlers wearing insulin pumps and CGMs; elementary kids bolusing for their meals at the table; teens together, away from their parents, talking about diabetes at school; parents trading tips for dealing with school; adults talking about the challenges they face in the workplace. Interspersed are world-renowned clinicians and researchers, who are sitting in the crowd and sharing their wisdom before they present at a scientific session. And all the food you're eating is carb-counted for you. Sound amazing? It is—and it's what happens at every Friends for Life conference.

Friends for Life conferences are organized by Children with Diabetes (CWD), a 501c3 nonprofit that I run. And they are exactly as I described above: the perfect place to meet others living with type 1, learn, and have an amazing experience.

There are other conferences, too—some large, some small held around the country all year long. JDRF chapters across the country hold one-day events featuring great speakers and vendors. They provide you with a great way to learn about diabetes care advances and see the latest diabetes care products available.

Another wonderful organization that holds conferences is called Taking Care of Your Diabetes (TCOYD). The group was founded by Steven V. Edelman, MD, an adult endocrinologist who has type 1 diabetes. TCOYD events include sessions for people with type 2 and type 1 diabetes and exhibits from diabetes care companies. They're fantastic one-day events that are held throughout the US.

Attending these events gives you a chance to hear from experts you would otherwise only read about, meet other parents who are facing similar challenges, and let your kids meet other kids—children with type 1 and their siblings—and realize that they are not alone. Attending a diabetes conference can be a life-changing experience for everyone. I highly recommend that you and your family make it a point to go to one, or more. Your diabetes care team will know about events in your community, and you can learn about Children with Diabetes conferences on its website.

18 Get Involved with the Diabetes Online Community

The term *diabetes online community* (DOC) refers to the large number of websites, blogs, and social media involved in all things related to diabetes. You will find incredible resources in the DOC, from scientific and medical education to support for your daily challenges.

But like all things online, there are some rules that can help you get the most from what the DOC offers. Here are my "Rules for Families" as they embark on their online journey:

- Just because it's on the Internet doesn't mean it's true.
- What works for one person may not work for you.
- Share what you find with your diabetes care team.
- Always look for the underlying science.
- The Internet is forever: be careful about the details you post.
- Don't take anything personally.

19   Maintain Your Privacy Online

I just mentioned a few rules for participating in the DOC. I want to expand upon one in particular because it really matters: the issue of privacy.

We've all seen posts in social media that we consider "oversharing": too much detail, photos that might be fine for immediate family but make friends cringe, and so on. In the world of diabetes—a world of chronic health care—you will have many opportunities to overshare. I would advise you to think very, very carefully about the kinds of things you post about your child with diabetes. Always think, "When my child with diabetes is an adult with diabetes, would they want to see what I am about to post?" And if you have even the slightest doubt, don't post.

You can also do what many of my friends have done: create a pseudonym for yourself and your child for all posts related to diabetes. This very effective tool lets you detail your child's diabetes experience while maintaining his anonymity.

20 Find Answers to Your Questions Online

If you have a nonurgent question about something diabetes-related and want to look for an answer online, look at reputable diabetes websites first before searching for answers on Facebook and other social media websites. Secondly, look for other good online resources, including the online version of the book *Understanding Diabetes* and the CWD website.

Most Facebook users are not medical professionals. (Those with medical backgrounds are good resources.) Most people on diabetes-related social media sites are parents or adults with type 1 diabetes. Keep in mind that while it's helpful to get input from other parents or adults with type 1 diabetes, your child's diabetes may respond differently than theirs does. I always recommend that families discuss things they've found online with their diabetes care team before making significant changes to their child's care.

21   Don't Do Nothing

As my friend Tom Karlya says, "Don't do nothing." Tom is well known in the type 1 diabetes community as Diabetes Dad for his maxim "Don't do nothing," which means that you should get involved in some way in the diabetes community. For some people, that means raising money for research. For others, it means helping out at summer camps or CWD conferences. For yet others, it means mentoring newly diagnosed families. It doesn't matter what you do—just do something.

22   Diabetes Care Is More Than HbA1c

As a parent, you might feel that your child's HbA1c is your report card. It's not. HbA1c is just one measure of how well you and your child are doing with regard to glucose management. With the advent of CGM, we've begun to understand the importance of glucose variability and range (the lowest low and the highest high) and the way these impact how someone with type 1 diabetes feels. Some in the field think that low variability might be even more important than a low HbA1c in reducing the risk for long-term complications. I always advise parents to view their child's HbA1c as one measure—but not the only measure—of their life with diabetes.

23 Siblings Matter

If you have other children, chances are they've been impacted by their sibling's diagnosis in ways you might not realize. Younger kids often hear "diabetes" and focus on the "di" part, worrying that their brother or sister is going to die. Older kids are often concerned about their sibling's health and family impact. They watched you worry in the days leading up to diagnosis, have seen you rush to the doctor or hospital, and now realize their family routine has forever changed. They don't often express this anxiety, but it's real and it's there. Teach them about diabetes as soon as you can: explain what diabetes is, show them glucose monitoring and insulin injections, and let them know that, while diabetes is now part of the family, their feelings and concerns are just as important as always. Make time to talk with your other kids about their feelings.

24 Prepare a Diabetes Emergency Kit

Remember the old adage, "The younger the child, the more stuff you need to take when you go out"? The same applies to a child with type 1 diabetes. You've got a glucose meter, test strips, and lancet; extra insulin pump supplies; backup syringe or insulin pen; emergency glucose and glucagon; perhaps even food and water. And that's just for the trip to visit a friend. But are you prepared for an emergency?

Every family should prepare a diabetes emergency kit. This kit should have everything you and your child need to survive for several days, including all your diabetes supplies (leave the insulin in the refrigerator), nonperishable food, water, copies of your diabetes prescriptions, batteries or chargers for pumps and sensors, and contact information for your diabetes care team. Put these items in a travel case or tote bag that is labeled and easy to find. Be sure to review its contents every couple of months.

25 Never Punish for Diabetes

Don't punish your child for diabetes—for off-kilter blood sugars or other unexpected results. The tools we use to care for type 1 diabetes today are truly amazing. With them, people with type 1 can accomplish anything. But even these tools have their limitations. People with type 1 still have high blood sugars and low blood sugars, and the reasons why might be known (more carbs than expected in food) or unknown (an underlying illness that you don't know is there). Thus it's not fair for a child, or an adult, to be punished for or made to feel bad about a blood sugar that's unexpected. If you keep this in mind, you'll remove a potential source of unnecessary stress from your family's life.

26 Understand Today's Science

The popular press often shares stories of a new "cure" for diabetes. That "cure" is almost always in mice, sometimes in rats, but never in humans. When those stories hit the news, your friends and family will surely reach out to you, excited to share. These stories are interesting, but we are not mice, and nothing that has "cured" a mouse has yet to be effective in humans. Some in the research community argue that the lack of success in translating any successful mouse therapy into humans argues against the use of these animals, but research using them continues. So expect to see more reports of cures for mice in the news. Lucky mice.

27 Mini-Dose Glucagon Rescue

One of the most important things you will learn from your diabetes care team is how to take care of your child's diabetes when she is sick. Illness changes diabetes management, making everything more challenging. If your child has a stomach illness, for example, treating low blood sugars with food of any kind can be a real challenge, if not impossible. But you may not be aware of an important tool in your toolbox: mini-dose glucagon rescue. Every parent should understand this very important tool. Basically, you mix up a glucagon rescue kit and deliver a small amount using an insulin syringe, not the glucagon syringe. The amount varies by age:

- 20 µg for kids two and under
- 10 µg per year of age for kids from two to fifteen (20 µg at age two, 30 µg at age three, and so on)
- 150 µg for kids fifteen or older

For more information, see the page on this topic on the Children with Diabetes website. Hamilton Health Sciences also includes details on how to draw up glucagon, with blood glucose levels in mmol/l instead of mg/dl.

And if you use a mini-dose rescue, be sure to renew your glucagon prescription immediately.

28   Cake Frosting Tubes for Treating Lows

There are lots of ways to treat low blood sugar, from juice and milk to candy to specially made glucose tablets. Glucose tablets are the most expensive solution (though they are not terribly expensive), but they offer the advantage of precise dosage and very long shelf life. Candy might be tempting to use, but then you are reinforcing lows with treats. Juice boxes also come in fixed volumes, but can bring their own family challenges if you have other kids who like to drink them. That could leave you without your low treatment—the juice box—when you need it the most.

One treatment to consider is small tubes of cake frosting or gel. The small decorating tubes offer a couple of advantages. First, they're very small and can fit in a parent's pocket or purse as well as in the glove compartment in a car. Second, they come in many flavors, helping to provide some variety. And third, you can squirt the gel into your child's mouth, which can help a lot at night when they're not quite awake. But be careful with dark colors because they can stain fabrics.

29   What to Do If You Mix Up Insulin Doses

At some point, most families give the wrong insulin dose to their child. If you give too little insulin, your child will have a higher-than-expected blood sugar. Dealing with that is easy— you give your child more insulin. But what if you give too much insulin? Or way too much insulin? That can happen if your child is on injections and you give the typical morning dose at night, or give a large dose of rapid-acting insulin instead of a large dose of long-acting insulin. Then what do you do?

If you realize the error immediately, don't panic. Even rapid-acting insulin analogs take fifteen to twenty minutes to begin working, so you have time to collect yourself. You have a few options.

First, your child can eat to cover the insulin. This might be a good time to have that hot fudge sundae with 150 grams of carbs that your child loves. As long as your child is hungry (and lots of insulin will make him hungry), this strategy usually works.

Second, if you've tried food and your child isn't hungry anymore or doesn't feel like eating, you can use your regular low blood sugar treatment. This might be a good time to try out mini-dose glucagon rescue as well.

Third, if these two strategies aren't working, contact your diabetes care team and ask for their advice. You can always go to an urgent care center or hospital and have your child treated with a glucose IV. This is the last resort of course, but it will work.

30   Additional Medicines to Have on Hand

It's harder to manage your diabetes when you're sick. It's especially challenging when your child has a stomach bug because she can have difficulty keeping low treatments down. I always recommend that families have on hand a prescription anti-nausea medication to help with nausea and vomiting. Your two options are ondansetron (generic for Zofran), originally developed to help cancer patients, and promethazine (generic for Phenergan). Both of these medications work well and can be the difference between treating a low blood sugar at home and taking your child to an emergency room. Check with your diabetes care team about which will work best for your child.

31   What to Keep in Your Car

In addition to whatever you normally take with you when you leave the house, you're now bringing diabetes care supplies. That usually means a glucose meter and strips; a lancing device and lancets; insulin, syringes or infusion sets; and low treatments. Which can you keep in your car to make it easier on yourself?

Glucose test strips and insulin are sensitive to temperature extremes, so they should not be kept in your car. You'll need to bring them with you each time you head out. Insulin, in particular, needs to be kept either refrigerated or at room temperature—not too cold, and not too hot—or it will not work well (or at all).

Lancing devices, lancets, syringes, and infusion sets can keep in most temperatures, so keeping spares in your car should be fine. If you keep some in your car, you might want to put them in a small bag with a note indicating the date you packed them.

You should always have some kind of low treatment and food in your car, so you'll need to choose products that can keep in both warm and cold weather. Glucose tablets work very well, as do certain candies, granola bars, and other packaged foods. Juice boxes can freeze, so they are probably not a good idea in parts of the country where the winter gets very cold. They can also get very hot in the summer sun. Check on these supplies periodically to be sure you have enough and that they are within their "best used by" dates.

32   Enjoy Birthdays and Holidays

When our daughter was young, diabetes care was very different than today. She took Regular and NPH insulin, and a blood glucose took 120 seconds to produce a result. We recorded blood sugars and insulin doses in a paper log. Birthdays and holidays often found her with blood sugars higher than usual, for all the reasons you might expect. She ate more than we planned, there were more carbs in the food than we thought, and the Regular insulin we injected took too long to work. That was life with type 1 in the late 1980s and 1990s.

When we brought those paper logs to our quarterly clinic visits, our daughter's doctor would make a note by those higher-than-expected readings. He'd write "Birthday" or "Party," and move on. He didn't fuss about those occasional highs, because he knew that enjoying life, enjoying the birthday or holiday, was much more important than worrying about the occasional high blood sugar. He was right then, and he's still right today.

2

Care Strategies for Babies through Preschool-Age Kids

Very young children with type 1 diabetes bring a couple of unique challenges—namely, determining when they are low and dealing with mealtime power struggles. Here are a few tips for making those challenges less challenging.

33 Preventing Lows Is Paramount

Managing type 1 diabetes is always a balancing act. You're trying to prevent both low and high blood sugars. Most medical professionals feel that preventing low blood sugars in very young children is more important than preventing high blood sugars, and most parents of very young kids fully agree. That doesn't mean that you should allow your child's blood glucose to run high. It just means that you should focus your efforts more on preventing lows than on preventing highs.

34 Is It a Tantrum or a Low Blood Sugar?

Perhaps the greatest challenge for parents of very young kids with type 1 diabetes is the child's inability to tell you exactly how he is feeling. This is most important for hypoglycemia. A temper tantrum in a two- or three-year-old can look a lot like a reaction to low blood sugar. The best advice I can offer parents of very young kids is to check blood sugar levels anytime your child exhibits any kind of behavioral problem, even a tantrum. The last thing you want to do is deal with the behavior and miss a low blood sugar.

If you can, get a continuous glucose monitoring (CGM) system for your child. A CGM offers immediate glucose values, sparing you from many finger-stick checks, and trend indicators to alert you to lows and highs in the near future.

35   Helping Your Child Feel Empowered

Even young kids with type 1 diabetes need to feel some sense of empowerment, which really comes down to having some say or choice in their care. Your child obviously doesn't have a choice in glucose monitoring or insulin injections (or pump sites), but you can give him an opportunity to choose which finger is used for a glucose check or where the next insulin injection is given (as long as you are practicing good site rotation practice). Even this small amount of choice can help reduce stress and give your child a sense of ownership and responsibility.

36   Avoiding Mealtime Power Struggles

Children don't always eat what parents want them to eat, and a young child with type 1 diabetes who has insulin on board in anticipation of a meal can be a source of considerable anxiety for parents. Many parents give in to the fear of an impending low blood sugar and offer their toddler dessert first, just to prevent a low. While pre-bolusing for meals is the best way to minimize the risk of post-meal high blood sugars, you may want to adopt a different strategy if you're faced with a fussy eater.

One option is to wait until your child finishes her meal to dose the full amount of mealtime insulin. This will help prevent post-meal lows, but it basically ensures that she will

31

have high blood sugar for hours after any meal with a sizeable amount of carbohydrates.

An alternative strategy is to give some of the mealtime insulin before the meal and the rest after you see how much she has eaten. This is a good compromise between diabetes control and parental sanity. And the good news is that your child will outgrow this temperamental eating phase, making mealtimes less stressful.

If you have given insulin and your child's blood sugar is in range or low, and he is absolutely refusing to eat the meal you have provided, consider giving him another option such as a small bowl of cereal with milk; a piece of toast with milk; or toast with cheese, peanut butter, or almond butter in order to prevent a low. This may not be what your dietitian or certified diabetes educator (CDE) would recommend, but as a parent you often have to do whatever it takes to get your child to eat.

For many people with type 1 diabetes, blood sugar spikes after breakfast are common. You can sometimes give the pre-breakfast insulin earlier, or give more insulin (a higher insulin-to-carbohydrate ratio) than at other meals. Consider a lower carbohydrate breakfast if possible, especially if your child's pre-breakfast blood sugar is elevated. This can help prevent a very high post-meal blood glucose.

You might find your child "sneaking" food occasionally. Try to determine why your child is eating extra food. Is his blood sugar low? Is he eating a lower protein diet? (Protein usually leaves you feeling full longer.) Is he just rebelling, being a child because he is a child? If he's old enough, discuss why he's eating extra and remind him that he needs insulin to cover extra carbohydrates. Be sure to discuss this with your diabetes team dietitian and/or psychologist. Generally, if you'd let your child eat more if he didn't have diabetes, then you need to find a way to let him eat more now that he does.

37   Have a System for Dosing Insulin

When kids with type 1 diabetes are young, Mom and Dad are responsible for dosing their insulin. If that responsibility is shared, it's a good idea to have a well-defined system in place for which parent is in charge of each dose. For example, Mom might be responsible for breakfast and bedtime doses, while Dad is responsible for overseeing lunch and dinner doses. Having this responsibility clearly defined helps prevent a missed dose, in which Mom thought Dad gave the insulin and Dad thought Mom gave the insulin—but in the end, no one did.

3

Care Strategies for Elementary-Age Kids

As kids grow into the elementary years, they will begin to spend time away from home, both at school and at their friends' homes. This can be scary for parents who are used to controlling their child's diabetes care. Here are some tips to help your child succeed and reduce parental anxiety.

38 Consider Getting Your Child a Mobile Phone

As a parent, it's normal for you to worry about your child when she's away from you, even if she's at school or a friend's home. It's also normal to worry more when type 1 diabetes is involved. Giving your child—even a child in elementary school—a mobile phone gives you the tool you need to keep in touch and help reduce that fear. I know many parents of young kids who provide their child with a mobile phone specifically to communicate diabetes care information. Their child will text or call a parent for guidance on bolusing insulin at lunch, report glucose levels when checked at school or at a friend's home, and generally keep parents informed. If you have the ability to get your child a mobile phone, I highly recommend that you do. (Of course, if you have other kids, that does set a precedent for early access to mobile phones.)

39 Building Safe Spaces at School

In the United States, kids with type 1 diabetes are entitled to the same level of care at school as they have at home, and they are entitled to participate in all school activities. Any school that receives public funding (including private schools) must comply with laws that provide for this. Parents are strongly encouraged to prepare a "Section 504 plan," outlining the specific care steps for their child. A 504 plan spells out when and where a child is permitted to check glucose levels, inject insulin (with or without adult supervision or assistance), have access to water and bathrooms, and implement any other care item that parents and the child's diabetes care team feel is important. These plans often specify that kids are permitted to check their blood sugar in the classroom to avoid time away from instruction, that they are allowed water and food if they feel the need, and that they are never to be left alone if they feel low. You'll find many sample 504 plans that you can tailor to your specific situation online at the ADA website and the CWD website.

It's very important to have diabetes care products in your child's classroom and in any other room she uses during the day (art room, music room, gym, and so on) in case her school experiences a lockdown event. Having emergency glucagon, food, and water available for your child could prevent adding a diabetes medical emergency to an already tense situation. And keeping those supplies, along with the diabetes care supplies, in a "to-go" type bag will make it easy to grab in case of evacuation.

The best resource to help kids at school is "Helping the Student with Diabetes Succeed: A Guide for School Personnel." You can download it from the National Institute of Diabetes and Digestive and Kidney Diseases (NIDDK) website.

40 Building Safe Spaces in the Neighborhood

Kids love to visit their friends' homes. For parents of kids with type 1 diabetes, that can be a source of anxiety. The best way to reduce that anxiety is to work with the parents of your child's friends to build a safe space at their homes. A simple way to do this is to get a small plastic container and fill it with whatever you use to treat lows, as well as some other food that you know your child will eat, just in case they are low and need food. A water bottle is also a good idea. Label it with your child's name so that everyone knows who and what it's for. Having these diabetes-low kits throughout your neighborhood will ensure that low treatments are always at hand in case your child goes low.

41 Having Fun During Trick-or-Treat

The bucket of candy that your child brings home from trick-or-treating presents a dilemma. On the one hand, you want your child to do anything they would have done without diabetes. On the other hand, the sugar in candy can be a challenge for insulin dosing. Families of kids with type 1 generally choose one of a few options:

- Let the child trick-or-treat, but trade the candy collected for something else.
- Donate the candy to a local children's hospital.
- Integrate the candy into lunches or snacks over the coming weeks. One treat a day, for example, is easy to accommodate.

Our family also changed what we gave out from candy to inexpensive toys, such as Halloween-themed pencils and bouncy balls. Kids seemed to appreciate those items because they lasted long after all their candy was consumed.

You'll face similar issues with other holidays that involve sweets, so it's best to decide on one approach and stick to it.

42   Managing Lunch at School

When your child heads off to the first full day of school, one of your biggest worries is how he will manage lunch. You're not there to estimate the amount of carbohydrates eaten and dose insulin accordingly. So what are you to do?

One option is to pack your child's lunch. That way you know exactly how many carbohydrates are in it. You can even write the number of carbs and the insulin dose on a piece of paper and put it in your child's lunch box or bag. That way, any adult who is there to help your child will know how to help decide how much insulin he should take for his food.

If your child wants to buy lunch at school, check with the school to see if they have nutrition information for each lunch offering. Schools typically post lunch menus weeks (if not months) in advance, so you can work with your child to plan when to buy meals that he likes and will eat.

Another option, if you have no school nurse and no one else is available to supervise your young child's lunchtime insulin dosing, is to consider giving a shot of Regular or NPH at breakfast to cover the carbohydrates eaten for lunch. The choice of insulin may depend on what time your child takes pre-breakfast insulin and what time lunch is held. While not ideal, this is one strategy to cover lunch. The options should be discussed with your diabetes team.

In the first days of each school year, you might find that your child's post-lunch blood sugar doesn't quite match what you expected based on the nutrient counts of both packed and bought lunches. That's to be expected. Going back to school is a time of stress and excitement. Plan to work with your child to make adjustments in the lunchtime insulin dose.

43   Insulin Dosing While Away from Home

When kids are away from parents and need insulin, whether at school or eating at a friend's house, parents have to find a way to help their child, or an adult, dose her insulin. Using an insulin pump can make this easier, since the insulin is already on their body (in the pump) and there's no need for another injection. For kids who don't use an insulin pump, your child (or an adult helper) will need to fill a syringe or dial up a dose in a pen and inject.

Schools that receive any public support are required by law to provide assistance for kids in their diabetes care. Often this is a school nurse or aide. Parents can meet with this adult helper to provide guidance on how their child takes her insulin.

When your child is away from home and school, you'll need to arrange for another adult to help younger kids and supervise older kids. While other parents can be anxious about needles and blood tests, you should be able to show them, calmly, how to easily help when needed. If your child has a mobile phone, you can call or text and supervise yourself.

44 Low Treatments Are Not Treats

As discussed earlier, a lot of people treat low blood sugars with juice, milk, or sugared soft drinks. These work great to increase blood sugar, but they are also regular food and can be seen as treats by young kids. I always advise parents of young kids to separate low treatments from regular food in some way. If you use glucose tablets, no one will mistake them for treats, but they are more expensive than alternatives. Some candy, like Skittles, work very well for treating lows and have even had a scientific poster presented on them. Again, the risk is that the candy will be seen as a treat, not a low treatment. Juice boxes are much the same.

If you decide to use candy or juice boxes to treat lows, don't include them in any meals. The goal is to separate diabetes care supplies from meals so that kids realize that their low treatments are just that: low treatments. Also, tell your other children that the low treatments are not to be consumed by anyone else, lest you find yourself out of them when you need them to treat a low blood sugar.

45 Sports

A child with type 1 is not prohibited from participating in any sport—even *scuba diving* is allowed. If your child wants to participate in a team sport, speak with the coach. Stress that your child is quite capable of playing unless her blood sugar is extremely high or low. You can help by providing your child's snacks and beverages and checking her blood sugar between innings, quarters, periods, or halftime. If your child wears a pump, make sure the pump is tucked in safely, but be prepared for an official/referee/umpire to tell your child to take off his "pager." You might want to check the rules of the sports association to make sure there are no issues with the pump or a medical identification product. (Some sports may say "no jewelry" for the safety of all players, and that includes kids with type 1 diabetes.)

Keep in mind that the weather may affect your child on the field as well. Some people with type 1 have highs when it is hot, lows when it is cold; others have the opposite. If you have specific questions about winter sports or endurance sports, consider contacting Riding on Insulin or Connected in Motion on their websites. For other questions, consider asking someone in the Facebook group "Type 1 Diabetic Athletes Group" (a group you would have to join).

46 Making Life Not About Diabetes

The very first tip in this book was about living life first, diabetes second. That's very easy to say but challenging to accomplish. Diabetes is often the first thing in every parent's mind. An example is when kids come home from school. Kids often say that the first thing they hear is, "How's your blood sugar?" That's making their life all about diabetes. Instead, they should hear, "How was your day?" Make life not about diabetes. You'll have plenty of time to discuss diabetes later.

4

Care Strategies for Tweens

The tween years, ages nine to twelve or so, are a transitional time. Kids typically still listen to their parents, haven't experienced the growth spurts and hormonal changes of puberty, and understand reasonably well about cause and effect and thus can participate actively in their diabetes care. But this is also the beginning of independence, so what you do in these years can have a lasting impact.

47 Get a Mobile Phone for Your Tween

While not every family feels that kids as young as nine or ten should have a mobile phone, I highly recommend that every tween with type 1 diabetes get one—even if the phone is to be used only for diabetes care discussions and messages. Just like with younger kids with diabetes who have mobile phones, you are always just a call or message away from being able to help your child. Beyond that, though, you're also giving your tween an important tool to use in developing confidence in taking over her own care, since she knows that she can reach out to you for confirmation of a decision or for help when she has a question.

48 Planning a Transition of Responsibility for Care

Everything you do as a parent is designed to help your child grow up to be a successful, independent adult. For parents of kids with type 1 diabetes, that includes helping them become self-sufficient in their diabetes care. It's never too early to discuss transitioning of this care with your child and with your child's diabetes team, but it's especially important to have begun this process by the time your child is a teen. That means you should begin planning the transition process while your child is a tween. While teens often know *how* to do diabetes care, they often forget to actually *do* their diabetes care (but adults do, too). A slow, well-planned transition—taking place over many years—is the best strategy for success.

49   Sleepovers for Tweens

As kids grow into the tween years, they often are involved in sleepovers at homes of friends. For parents of tweens with type 1 diabetes, that means blood glucose checks before dinner and before sleep, as well as insulin-dosing before dinner. Most tweens can assume responsibility, on occasion, for these diabetes care tasks, and with cell phones in the hands of tweens, parents can communicate directly with their tween to help as needed.

Even if you're anxious about your tween being away for an evening sleepover, letting her go is an important step in helping her learn how to care for herself. And even if her diabetes care isn't as good as it would have been at home, you're helping her become confident in her care, and you're showing her that her diabetes won't limit what she can do.

5

Care Strategies for Teens

Oh, the teen years. You may have heard about how challenging diabetes care is during the teen years. For some teens, that's the case, but it needn't be a time of turmoil—at least not in terms of diabetes. Here are some thoughts to help your family thrive during the teen years.

50   Sharing versus Not

The teen years are all about your child finding his own way in the world. That includes diabetes care. And one way this is reflected is in how much he shares with you about his life. That, too, includes diabetes care.

You might have been involved in every glucose check and insulin dose when he was twelve, but that's not going to be the case when he's sixteen, much less when he's eighteen. You'll need to work with your teen to establish rules about how much of his diabetes care you remain involved in as he grows through his teen years.

51   Remaining Engaged as a Parent

A considerable body of scientific evidence shows that children whose parents who remain engaged in their diabetes care as they grow into adulthood have better outcomes as adults. Basically, this means that parents need to stay involved in their child's diabetes care—but you should scale it back gradually rather than hand it over to your child all at once as she grows into the teen years. There are many ways to remain engaged, and exactly what you do will depend on your relationship with your child. Some parents offer to check blood sugars for their kids on weekend mornings, giving them time to sleep longer. Some help with carbohydrate counting during family meals.

Some assist with filling prescriptions. It doesn't matter what you do as a parent. What matters is that you are doing something to provide support to your child as she grows into adulthood.

52 Peers Really Matter

Whether you like it or not, your teen's peers are much more important to her than you are as parents. As a result, your teen's peers can have a profound impact on her diabetes care. You can help by encouraging your teen to share her diabetes with her closest friends and be there to help explain type 1 diabetes and its care, if needed. You want your child's peers to be supportive and understanding. You also want them to understand the importance of checking blood sugar and taking insulin so that your child isn't embarrassed or anxious about doing these things.

53 Sex, Drugs, and Alcohol

Your teen will be exposed to sex, drugs, smoking, and alcohol—whether you realize it or not. Type 1 diabetes complicates all of these issues, and it's vitally important for teens with type 1 to know the medical facts about these issues because the consequences are much more serious for them than for their friends without type 1.

Let's start with sex—specifically for girls. The issue is about pregnancy, and the importance of always planning a pregnancy. Women with type 1 diabetes can have a safe and healthy pregnancy and baby, but it needs to be planned to ensure the best outcome. Teenage girls with type 1 diabetes should be discussing birth control with their diabetes care team without a parent in the room. I realize that some parents will be extremely uncomfortable with this recommendation, but the fact is that teens are often sexually active before parents realize it, and a girl with type 1 diabetes should never have an unplanned pregnancy. Ensuring the latter is more important than anything else. The JDRF offers an excellent guide on pregnancy with type 1 diabetes on its website.

Teens need to know how alcohol affects their bodies. Again, teens are often exposed to alcohol long before parents might suspect, and knowing what alcohol does in someone with type 1 diabetes can mean the difference between life and death. Of particular concern with alcohol is that the symptoms of a low blood sugar are often the same as being drunk, so it's vitally important that your teen (and young adult) wear a medical identification product, either a bracelet or necklace, that states Type 1 Diabetes. Should something unexpected happen, first responders will look for a bracelet or necklace and will know that your child has type 1.

54   Teen Girls and Menstrual Cycles

When your daughter has her period and has diabetes, she will have higher blood sugars. It's simple: the hormone fluctuations that girls experience cause blood sugars to increase. There are ways to help, such as having alternate basal patterns on a pump, or using temporary basal increases. If your teen uses injections, you can add a little extra insulin for meals. Be sure to work with your teen's diabetes care team on exactly how much to adjust. Above all, remember it's possible she'll be grumpy because of the fluctuating hormones, so it's not an ideal time for parents to become frustrated with high blood sugars.

55   Helping Teens Remember to Take Their Insulin

I've mentioned the importance of pre-bolusing. Even more important is simply taking insulin for meals. During the teen years, kids are busier than ever and often have to get up earlier than they would like to get to school. Forgetting to take mealtime insulin is easy given this situation. One way you can help is to put a small note on the inside of their bedroom door that says, "Bolus for Breakfast." It's a gentle reminder that just might make a difference when your teen is running late on school mornings.

56   Look for College Scholarships

Several organizations provide college scholarships for kids with type 1 diabetes. Ask your diabetes care team about funders in your area. One national organization, the Diabetes Scholars Foundation, offers several annual scholarships for incoming freshman who have type 1 diabetes. This scholarship program is extremely competitive, with a couple thousand students submitting applications every year. You can learn more on the Diabetes Scholars Foundation website. Several other organizations, including Team Type 1, the Scott and Kim Verplank Foundation, and the College Diabetes Network, offer college scholarships as well. See their websites for details.

57   Driving Is Special

A driver's license is the gateway to freedom for teenagers and the source of unending anxiety for parents—especially parents of teens with type 1 diabetes. Several studies show that drivers with type 1 have an increased risk for automobile accidents, with low blood sugar the likely cause. Teens with type 1 who drive assume extra responsibility for their diabetes care, which means always checking blood glucose levels before driving, having rapid-acting glucose within reach, and never driving when low. Using a CGM is a very good idea, because a finger-stick glucose reading in the target range at the start of a drive can change to a low very quickly while driving. This milestone offers you a great opportunity to help your teen assume more responsibility for his own care. Take advantage of it and establish clear diabetes care rules before he begins driving.

One additional note: Most states in the US require disclosure of diabetes. Failure to do so can result in both the loss of a driver's license and the loss of car insurance in the event of an accident. I always recommend disclosing diabetes. You can learn more about the laws in each state from the ADA website.

58   Stepping Back as a Parent

When your child with type 1 heads off to college, your involvement in her diabetes care will rapidly decrease and might quickly end. You'll need to work with your teen to develop a family transition plan of care so she is capable of diabetes self-care before heading off to school. You can prepare for this day by gradually stepping back during the last year of high school. Two key new responsibilities that your child will assume will be arranging her own medical care and ordering her diabetes care supplies. Teaching her about health insurance coverage, prescriptions, how to order supplies, and how to schedule medical appointments while she is still in high school is vitally important. Teach her how before she needs to do it on her own.

6

Care Strategies for College and Beyond

As teens approach college, parents can be understandably anxious about how well their teen will do on her own. I've often heard parents of older teens say that they plan to move into their child's dorm room in college to make sure that she takes care of her diabetes. Thankfully, I don't know of any parent who has followed through on that feeling.

59 Setting Your Child Up for Success in College

Few events are more stressful for parents of kids with type 1 diabetes than the day the kids head off to college. For the first time in their lives, college kids with type 1 diabetes are essentially on their own. Your primary goal as a parent—other than trying not to show your anxiety—is to help your college student with type 1 succeed in life, as you would do if your child didn't have diabetes. Some ways to do this include ordering extra diabetes care supplies ahead of time (you might need to convince your insurance company that this is necessary) so he has months of items to begin with; ensuring that he has a medical identification product that he will wear; identifying a local pharmacy that can fill his prescriptions (a twenty-four-hour pharmacy is always best); making sure that his roommate and resident advisor are aware of his diabetes; and asking your current diabetes care team for suggestions about care where your child is going. You should also establish ground rules about communicating diabetes care issues. This will be especially important to reduce parental anxiety if you've been used to monitoring your child's diabetes closely in recent years.

60 Finding Support in College

Two national organizations, the College Diabetes Network and Students with Diabetes, offer organized support for college students with type 1 diabetes, through their network of chapters on college campuses. Their chapters bring knowledge of the local community, including nearby diabetes care teams and the all-important nearest 24/7 pharmacy.

These organizations are great resources for college students and their families. If your child's school doesn't have a chapter, both groups offer ways to start one. (And you can find helpful information on their websites.)

61 Caring Might Not Be Sharing

At some point, your child will decide that he doesn't want to share his diabetes with you anymore. If you've been working on a transition to independence for many years, you'll reach this event gradually and you'll be ready for it. If you haven't been working on the transition . . . well, this moment can catch you by surprise. Regardless, know that this day is coming, and know that it is an important milestone in your child's maturation into a self-sufficient adult. Though it can be painful for you, this is the ultimate goal for your child.

62 Fostering Independence Means Allowing Failure

I've mentioned transitioning responsibility multiple times, and will again because it's very important. Transitioning is about fostering independence, and like in all things, that means giving your child permission to try and fail. In diabetes care, failure can mean many things, including experiencing unexpected high and low blood sugars. Giving your child permission to try and fail (and treat a low or high) is critically important in helping him to learn how to succeed. There will come a time when you must step back and merely advise, allowing your child to make a decision, even if that decision isn't what you would do. That's how we all learn.

63 Trust but Verify

As you transition responsibility for diabetes care tasks to your child, it's very important to remain involved. I call this "Trust But Verify." This "Trust But Verify" policy can take many forms. As an example, you can agree to review blood glucose meter readings, CGM tracings, and boluses on an insulin pump daily while your child is in high school, weekly during her first year of college, and monthly thereafter. Use that review as an opportunity to help with decision-making and problem-solving skills, rather than as a way to "catch" your child in a mistake. Remember: Your goal is to help your child learn to make good diabetes care decisions, and you'll achieve that goal better and sooner by providing positive, not negative, reinforcement. And your child will participate more readily if you're supporting her rather than berating her.

64 Adult Diabetes Care Is Very Different from Pediatric Care

Young adults with type 1 diabetes are often shocked by the change in how they're treated when they go to their first "adult" diabetes care clinic visit. Gone is the often years-long relationship with their pediatric diabetes care team. Gone is the deep understanding of type 1 diabetes. And gone are Mom and Dad accompanying them to the visit.

Instead, young adults with type 1 find themselves in an office filled mostly with adults with type 2 diabetes, and may find a care team that doesn't understand the intensive management required for type 1 diabetes. I know many young adults who returned from their first adult clinic visit shaken by the experience. My advice is to realize that adult care is different and to visit more than one adult endocrine office (assuming you have options) before making a decision on whom to see for your child's adult care. You're looking for a diabetes care team that values your perspective and understands that type 1 diabetes is different from the much more common type 2 diabetes.

65 The Importance of Health Insurance

It goes without saying that people with type 1 diabetes should have health insurance, but I'll say it anyway. Many studies show that people with diabetes, regardless of type, who do not have health insurance have worse outcomes than people who have health insurance. For young people with type 1 diabetes, the need for health insurance might weigh into decisions about career choice. It's certainly something to consider for parents and teens as they begin to plan for their future.

66 Friends in Place of Parents

One of the hardest things to do as a parent of a child with type 1 diabetes is to step back from being involved in your child's care. You worry about whether they will be safe, especially with regard to their diabetes care. One way to make this transition to independence easier is to help your child's friends learn about type 1 so they can be there when you are not. Encourage your child to confide in her best friend or friends and teach them about diabetes care, including how to check blood sugar or read a CGM display, how to disconnect an insulin pump, and when to call for help.

7

Care Strategies for All Ages

There are a few care strategies that can make a real difference in metabolic and quality of life outcomes for children of all ages. Adopting these strategies and integrating them into your child's life are easy, so there's no reason not to do so. Here are my suggestions.

67 Manage Important Information

Type 1 diabetes is, above all, an information management challenge. You use blood glucose data, estimates of carbohydrates in food, planned exercise, levels of stress, and whatever else impacts blood sugars to decide how much insulin to dose at a given time. This is really complicated. However, the more data you have, the better decisions you can make, and the most important piece of data you use is blood glucose values.

If you're using finger-stick glucose monitoring as your only tool to gather this data, checking your child a lot of times per day is very important. Before CGM, people with type 1 diabetes would often check ten or more times per day. Regardless of how many times per day you check, data from the T1D Exchange demonstrates that more frequent daily glucose monitoring results in lower HbA1c results, across all ages.

68 Know How to Use Different Kinds of Insulin

Today, most people with type 1 diabetes in the US use insulin analogs. These are engineered insulins that are designed to work either more quickly than human insulin or last longer than human insulin. If your child uses an insulin pump, he uses only a rapid-acting insulin analog. If he takes insulin in multiple daily injections, he uses both a rapid-acting analog to cover his meals and a long-acting insulin analog to cover his basal insulin needs. But there are two other types of insulin you should know about and understand: Regular and NPH.

Before insulin analogs, people who needed insulin used Regular, a short-acting insulin, and NPH, a longer-acting basal insulin. While many studies show better outcomes using analogs (especially a reduction in hypoglycemia), Regular and NPH insulin are used by more people worldwide than analogs, mostly due to cost: Regular and NPH are significantly less expensive than analogs. In the US, Regular and NPH do not require a prescription, a fact that can become important if your child is away from home or loses his insulin and needs to replace it quickly.

Given their widespread and easy availability, it's worth discussing how to use Regular and NPH in an emergency with your child's diabetes care team.

69   Bolus Well before Meals

One of the best ways to achieve an HbA1c in your child's target range is to give her mealtime insulin well before she eats a meal. A study published in 2010 concluded that pre-meal boluses need to be taken twenty minutes before eating to prevent a large rise in post-meal glucose levels.

Injecting insulin twenty minutes before eating can be a challenge for parents of a young kid because you might not be sure how much she will eat. However, you can give some insulin to get it working on reducing blood glucose levels, and that will help reduce post-meal high blood sugar readings. Older kids should get in the habit of pre-bolusing. It makes a big difference.

70 Consider an Insulin Pump

Insulin pumps offer an alternative to injections, but they are more expensive and require more work, too. So why do people use them? Because they make diabetes care easier and can help provide better health outcomes.

If you're new to type 1 diabetes, adding an insulin pump might seem like more than you can handle. But insulin pumps today are very easy to use and offer some significant advantages over injections, especially for kids. Most importantly, insulin pumps can deliver very small amounts of insulin very precisely—something you cannot do with a syringe or an insulin pen. For small kids, insulin pumps are often the only way to deliver the correct insulin dose without diluting insulin.

Another big advantage of insulin pumps is that the insulin is always with you. If your child uses a syringe or a pen, he might forget it when he goes out. Since the insulin pump is attached to your child, he can't forget it. (Of course, you need to be sure that he has enough insulin in the pump, but the pump will alert you when you need to refill it.)

71 If You Pump, Know How to Untether

"Untethering" refers to using both an insulin pump and injections at the same time. It sometimes refers to pump users who switch between using a pump and using injections, depending upon what they're doing. For example, if your child uses an insulin pump and is planning a weekend at the beach, she might want to leave the pump at home—away from the sand, salt, and sea—and use injections. There are several strategies for "untethering," and your child's diabetes care team can help her figure out what works for her. The CWD website features a good introduction to this subject by Dr. Steven Edelman.

72 Continuous Sensors Change Everything

I am convinced that the single biggest advance in diabetes care technology since insulin analogs in the 1990s is the advent of CGM. CGM systems use a small sensor, inserted under the skin, to provide a glucose reading every five minutes and to provide trajectory information about where the glucose reading is heading. This is an amazing improvement over finger-stick glucose readings; it is like the difference between a still photograph and a movie.

CGM systems provide alarms to warn of a low (or impending low) blood sugar or a high blood sugar, giving parents and kids a chance to treat a low before it becomes serious. This is very important, especially for parents caring for kids at night.

73   Share Your CGM Data

CGM systems allow you to view your child's glucose data remotely, using one of several technologies. This remote viewing feature is an incredible advance and should be used by everyone who has a CGM. And it's reason enough to get your child a CGM if he doesn't already have one.

Remote monitoring lets parents keep an eye on their child's blood glucose value when they're not together, such as when the child is at school or at a friend's house. As a parent, having this knowledge can greatly reduce the anxiety of not knowing.

If you use a CGM and don't have remote monitoring, ask your CGM provider for a way to get it, or check out Nightscout's website.

74   Stick with One or Two Fingers

Diabetes educators often recommend that you rotate spots for fingerstick blood glucose monitoring. I'm going to suggest something different: pick one or two spots on your child and stick with them for months at a time. The outer pad of the ring finger is an ideal location because it's not involved in precision touching. By using the same spot or spots over and over, that area will build up a small callus, and the spot will be less sensitive. Since blood glucose meters require so little blood (even with the callus), you'll be able to get enough blood to do a glucose check. After a couple of months, you can change the location, the sensation will return, and the callus will go away.

75   Alternate Site Blood Glucose Monitoring

Some kids hate using their fingertips for blood glucose monitoring. The good news is that you don't have to use fingers. You can use alternative sites, such as the side of the hand or the forearm. Most glucose meters support the use of alternative sites, but you need to bear two things in mind. First, glucose levels in alternative sites won't be exactly the same as fingertips, especially when glucose levels are changing rapidly. Second, rubbing the alternative site a bit before checking can help you get the right amount of blood more easily. Be sure to speak with your diabetes care team if you use alternative site checking.

76   Injection Site Rotation Really Matters

While I suggested using the same spot for finger sticks for months at a time, the same doesn't apply to insulin site injections or insulin pump infusion sites. Your child's diabetes team will have taught you about site rotation. I can't emphasize enough how important good site rotation habits are. Your child will be taking injections for years, perhaps his entire life. Site rotation is essential to maintain the health of the skin and subdermal tissue. There are many strategies to help you with site rotation. Ask your care team for suggestions. You can also check out a great product called Tartoos, temporary tattoos for proper injection site management.

77 Don't Use a Public Bathroom for Diabetes Care

Let's be very clear on this: public bathrooms are not clean and should never be used for diabetes care. When you're out at a restaurant, check blood sugar and inject or bolus at the table. You can be discreet enough that no one should notice or care.

Cleanliness isn't your only concern. If you relegate diabetes care tasks to bathrooms, you're sending your child a message that diabetes is something to be ashamed of or has to be hidden. Don't do that. Check and inject in public.

78 You Can Inject through Clothing

Let's say you've checked your child's blood glucose at a restaurant and you're ready for the pre-meal injection (well ahead of the meal, remember?). But it's winter, and your child is covered, head to toe, with clothes. You don't want to go to the bathroom (see above), but you need to make an injection. What do you do?

Inject right through your child's clothing.

Yes, you can inject through clothing. A study in the prestigious journal *Diabetes Care* was published in 1996 on just that topic.

79   Check Blood Ketones, Not Urine Ketones

When the body burns fat instead of glucose for energy, it produces a byproduct called "ketones." When someone with type 1 diabetes doesn't take enough insulin, their body will begin to use fat for energy. That is a serious problem and can lead to a very dangerous and life-threatening condition called diabetic ketoacidosis. That's why everyone with type 1 diabetes needs to know how to check for ketones.

Ketones can be measured in urine, but they can also be measured in blood, and blood is the much better way to check for ketones. The ketones in urine could have been produced hours before you check for them. When you check blood for ketones, you know the ketone level at that moment.

When kids are ill, it's much easier to check blood ketones than urine ketones—your child doesn't have to get out of bed.

Plus, kids really don't pee on command, but you can always get a drop of blood.

Two companies make combined blood glucose/blood ketone meters: Abbott Diabetes Care, which makes the Precision Xtra, and Nova Biomedical, which makes the Nova Max Plus. Regardless of which meter you use to measure blood glucose, every family living with type 1 diabetes should have one of these blood ketone meters on hand.

Ask your diabetes care team about when to contact them if your child develops ketones. Very high ketones can be a sign of diabetic ketoacidosis, which requires emergency medical care.

80   Be Open to Type 2 Medications

In the past several years, drug companies have developed a number of new therapies for adults with type 2 diabetes that can also have a positive impact on people with type 1 diabetes. Two classes of drugs have shown potential and have been studied in adults with type 1.

The first class are called GLP-1 agonists and have the trade names Victoza (liraglutide), Byetta/Bydureon (exenatide), and Trulicity (dulaglutide), to name a few. These drugs are injected daily or weekly and aim to control blood glucose levels by slowing the absorption of food after a meal and suppressing glucagon secretion, which helps to keep post-meal blood sugars from spiking. These drugs also make you feel full faster, helping people lose weight.

The second class are called SGLT-2 inhibitors and have the trade names Invokana (canagliflozon), Farxiga (dapagliflozin), and Jardiance (empagliflozin), among others. These drugs stop the kidneys from reabsorbing as much glucose as normal, resulting in the body urinating out a lot of glucose. They can help lower blood glucose all day long and can also help you lose weight.

Each of these classes of drugs brings benefits and risks, especially the SGLT-2 inhibitors, which can cause euglycemic ketoacidosis, a potentially very serious condition. Use of these drugs in people with type 1 is off-label, but is allowed if you and your diabetes care team think the benefits are worth the risks for your older child.

81   Go Ahead and Use the Hot Tub

You may have seen a warning sign beside a hot tub advising people with diabetes not to use it. That doesn't apply to your child. The warning is aimed at older adults with type 2 diabetes who might have loss of sensation due to neuropathy, a potential complication from years of high blood sugars. Children with type 1 diabetes can enjoy pools and hot tubs, just like other kids.

One word of caution: Insulin can be absorbed much faster while sitting in a hot tub, or even during a hot shower, resulting in low blood sugar. Be mindful of that and check your child's blood sugar often if she's enjoying a hot tub.

82   Be Mindful of Double Diabetes

Kids with type 1 diabetes are not immune from modern life, and modern life includes the risk of developing type 2 diabetes—even for kids with type 1 diabetes. Be mindful of the strategies to prevent type 2 diabetes, including eating healthy, not becoming overweight, and exercising often. These are important for everyone, and especially important for kids with type 1 diabetes.

83   Get Your Whole Family Checked for Celiac

Celiac is an autoimmune disease in which exposure to gluten, a protein in wheat and some other grains, causes damage to the small intestine and can lead to serious health issues. Recent studies estimate that one in ten people with type 1 diabetes also has celiac disease. As a result, everyone with type 1 diabetes should be screened for celiac. I also recommend that everyone in the family be screened, since I know many families in which one of the parents has celiac and the child has type 1 diabetes.

Living with celiac requires eating a gluten-free diet, which has become much easier in recent years with the rapid proliferation of prepackaged gluten-free foods.

84 Traveling Domestically with Diabetes

In the United States, people with diabetes are allowed to bring diabetes care supplies, including liquids, onto an airplane. For families who have a kid with type 1 diabetes, that means carrying insulin as well as juice boxes for treating lows, and water bottles to help with a high blood sugar. You'll need to declare these as medical supplies to the TSA screener. You can find more details on the Transportation Security Administration website.

85 Traveling Internationally with Diabetes

For families who travel internationally, the rules for what you can carry onto a plane are not the same as they are in the United States. Some suggestions:

- Make sure that your child with type 1 diabetes is wearing a medical identification product of some kind (a bracelet or necklace). This is important in the event your child is sick or injured, as it will help first responders and medical personnel recognize that your child has type 1 diabetes.

- Carry with you current prescriptions for all diabetes medications and products (insulin(s), glucose meter, syringes, lancets, and so on).
- Bring the full contact information for your child's diabetes care team.
- Always carry all diabetes care products with you. Never check any medical items.
- Bring enough supplies to last at least twice as long as you are planning to be away.

Check with your health insurance plan to find out what they will cover in case of an emergency while you are outside the country. If you find your coverage to be lacking, you can purchase reasonably priced travel medical insurance to cover your family.

Ask your diabetes care team if they can provide you with contact information for a diabetes care team near where you are traveling. That can come in very handy in case you have a medical emergency while you are away from home.

86 Don't Store Insulin in Hotel Refrigerators

The small refrigerators found in hotel rooms are no place to store insulin. Their temperature regulation is not like your home refrigerator, and you might find yourself with frozen, and thus useless, insulin if you store your child's insulin in it. Insulin can be stored safely at room temperature for a month.

If you're concerned about the temperature of your insulin while on vacation, consider getting something like a FRIO Insulin Cooling Case.

87 Reminders Before Heading Out on a Trip

In the haste of heading out the door for a trip, it's easy to forget items you meant to bring. You can't forget your child's diabetes care supplies, however. An easy way to help you remember these supplies is to tape a list of everything you need to bring with you to the inside of the door through which you leave. Prepare that list well before you leave and put it on the door as a final reminder before you head off on your trip. You'll be glad you did.

8

Final Thoughts

We've covered a lot of tips so far, and each can help you and your child live well with type 1 diabetes. What follows are some final thoughts that I think are important.

88   Type 1 Is Hard

Even on days when your child's blood sugar levels are in range, caring for type 1 diabetes is hard work. And on days when you are doing everything right and nothing is working, it's even harder. It's OK to acknowledge that. In fact, you *should* acknowledge that. The fact is, type 1 is tougher than most people realize, and certainly tougher than anyone who doesn't live with it can ever fully understand. Let your child know this by saying things like, "I know this is hard. We'll do this together." You'll be surprised at how much this can help.

89   How to Discuss Complications

Fear is not a good motivator for behavior change. Even knowing that, many parents warn their child with type 1 diabetes that they will go blind, lose a limb, or have their kidneys fail if they don't take care of themselves. As a parent, I think this is a terrible approach to helping a child with type 1 diabetes learn to take care of himself. Our goal as parents has to be to help our child understand that he will feel better and do better by participating in his diabetes care, rather than threatening him with long-term complications if he doesn't. The bottom line: unless your child brings up complications, focus on positive care decisions and leave the discussions about complications to your child's diabetes care team.

90 Don't Threaten Using the Problems of Others

I've heard of parents who threaten to take their child to meet an older adult with diabetes (not specifying which type) who has lost a limb due to diabetes-related nerve damage as a way of motivating them to take care of themselves. This is a terrible idea. Younger kids will just get scared, teens will be ashamed of themselves and you, and you won't accomplish your goal.

Older adults with type 1 diabetes grew up in a very different time and with very different tools to help them manage diabetes. Their experiences are fundamentally different from those of our kids today, just as other experiences from the past aren't necessarily relevant today.

Here's wisdom from Jill Weissberg-Benchell, PhD, CDE, a well-known psychologist who works with kids with diabetes:

"Frightening a child to 'teach them a lesson' never works. It makes them frightened. It makes them feel ashamed, and it guarantees that they will never be honest with their parents when they have struggles for fear that they will be shamed and blamed again. It makes sure that there is no collaboration between the parent and child in working together to deal with the ups and downs of life with diabetes."

81

91   Understand the Data on Complications

Historically, people with type 1 diabetes had a significant risk for developing long-term complications, including blindness, kidney damage, and nerve damage leading to amputation. The key word in that sentence is "historically." Beginning in the 1980s, with the advent of home blood glucose monitoring, and later in the early 1990s, with the knowledge gained from a study known as the Diabetes Control and Complications (DCCT), improvements in care resulted in a decline in the incidence of long-term complications. In the mid-2000s, studies from Sweden reported a dramatic reduction in the incidence of complications in people who had lived for decades with type 1 diabetes. Additional studies from Scandinavia and other countries, including the United States, all show the same thing: the incidence of serious complications is declining, and lifespans for people with type 1 diabetes are increasing.

92   What's Changed and Why It's Important

So what's changed that has resulted in the decline in the incidence of complications? Several things, including:

• Home blood glucose monitoring, which became widespread in the 1980s, provides accurate data insulin dosing and guidance on care decisions.

- Insulin analogs, both rapid-acting and long-acting, which provide more predictable action (long-acting analogs) and much faster onset of action (rapid-acting analogs).

- Insulin pumps, which allow micro-dosing of insulin and allow for variations in delivery throughout the day.

- Continuous glucose monitoring (CGM), a breakthrough technology that provides minute-by-minute insight into both glucose value and trajectory, offering predictions of future glucose values for the first time.

- Low-power wireless communications, which allow CGM devices to communicate with parents and others, offering remote support to people living with type 1 diabetes.

- Drugs to help with blood pressure that protect kidneys.

- New medicines and treatments for retinal bleeding that help repair minor problems and forestall major problems.

All of these advances combine to help people living with type 1 diabetes remain healthy far beyond what was possible even one generation ago.

93 People with Type 2 Are Our Allies

Most people don't know the difference between type 1 and type 2 diabetes, and that can be the source of a lot of misunderstanding. It's the basis for comments like, "So, you must have given your child a lot of sugar, right?" People say this because of a misperception, portrayed often in the public press, that diabetes (meaning type 2) is caused by overeating, and with that misperception often comes a tendency to blame the person for their diabetes.

Emerging science is hinting that there is much more to type 2 diabetes than simple lifestyle choices. Research into the gut microbiome, for example, hints at gut bacteria differences as potential causes for being overweight and obesity, key risk factors in developing type 2 diabetes.

Regardless of the underlying cause, we must stop blaming people for developing type 2 diabetes and remove the stigma associated with that blame.

We in the type 1 community live with the same challenges that people in the type 2 community do—low blood sugars, high blood sugars, medication, careful eating. Let's treat them as the allies they are.

94   Your Doctor Works for You

Always remember that your doctor and your diabetes team work for you. You don't work for them. Your diabetes team is in place to advise you and your child about the best way to take care of your child's diabetes within the context of her life and her goals. If you are not comfortable with how that relationship is going, or if you don't feel that the team is taking your child's concerns or goals seriously, or if your team won't consider new technology or strategies, be willing to find a new care team that will. As a parent, you have precious few years to help your child grow into a happy, healthy, and successful adult. Don't waste any of those years with a health care team that isn't fully on your side.

95 Ordering Supplies Can Be Challenging

More and more insurance companies are requiring their customers to use mail order pharmacies for medications. Often, diabetes care products fall into this category. If you use a mail order pharmacy for your supplies, be very careful not to run out. Shipping times can be delayed, or your supplier might need to verify coverage with your diabetes care team. It's a good idea to ask your child's doctor to prescribe enough of each diabetes care product to account for errors, loss, and damage. That way you're not short right before your new order arrives.

96 Write Down Your Child's Diabetes Care Data

Modern diabetes care involves a lot of data, and it's not just blood glucose values. If your child uses an insulin pump, he has basal rates, insulin-to-carbohydrate ratios, and correction factors programmed into the pump. Even if he doesn't use a pump, he uses that data when injecting basal and mealtime insulin. It's a good idea to write down that data and keep it in your child's diabetes emergency kit, just in case he experiences a catastrophic device failure or a natural disaster.

97 Your Child Might Need Additional Help

Sometimes, in spite of the best efforts of parents and diabetes care teams, a child with type 1 diabetes might also need real help with their mental health. If you find your child is in that situation, your first resource is the psychologist on your child's diabetes care team. Don't wait if you think your child might need help.

If your local team doesn't have the resources, or if your child needs more assistance, look into the inpatient mental health hospitals in the US that have programs specifically designed for teens with type 1 diabetes who have mental health needs. The best known is Cumberland Hospital for Children and Adolescents in Virginia. There are others, too. Your diabetes care team can advise you.

98 Get Involved in Research

As I've said for many years, all the money in the world in the hands of the most brilliant researchers in the world cannot make a difference in the lives of people living with type 1 diabetes if we, the families living with it, do not participate in research. I feel that participating in research is a moral obligation for all of us in the type 1 diabetes community, and I strongly encourage parents to ask their care teams about research in their local community as well as national and international research efforts in which they can participate. And note that siblings can participate in some trials, especially those that are investigating risk factors for developing type 1 diabetes like TrialNet. See their website for details.

99 Avoid Being the "Diabetes Police"

We've all met members of the "diabetes police." These are the people who tell you what you can't eat, ask you why you didn't check your blood sugar, and generally insert themselves into your care without your permission. Parents of kids with type 1 diabetes walk a fine line between parenting and being the diabetes police. The differences are subtle but important.

Parenting involves guiding and teaching. Members of the diabetes police often focus on criticizing choices that don't match their idealized vision of what diabetes is about. As your child grows up, you must be mindful to avoid being perceived as the diabetes police.

100 Great Books for Your Diabetes Library

If you're looking for a comprehensive book about caring for type 1 diabetes, there are several great books from which you can choose. I have two recommendations that stand out above all others:

Understanding Diabetes by H. Peter Chase, MD, and David M. Maahs, MD, PhD, published by the Children's Diabetes Foundation of Denver, Colorado. This book is typically called "The Pink Panther Book" because the Pink Panther is used throughout to portray someone with diabetes. Drs. Chase and Maahs have written the easiest-to-understand book about caring for type 1 diabetes in children and young adults.

Type 1 Diabetes in Children, Adolescents and Young Adults by Ragnar Hanas, MD. Dr. Hanas, a world-renowned pediatric endocrinologist from Sweden, has written the most complete book about caring for children with type 1 diabetes. The details in this book could serve as a textbook for physicians, yet the text is accessible to everyone. There are several versions, so be sure to get the one aimed at people who live in your country.

There are several other exceptional books (in alphabetical order) that are worth having in your diabetes library as well:

Balancing Diabetes: Conversations About Finding Happiness and Living Well by Kerri Sparling. The author is the voice of Six Until Me, one of the most widely read blogs in the diabetes community. *Balancing Diabetes* is a great collection of wisdom from Sparling and others who live with type 1.

Breakthrough: Elizabeth Hughes, the Discovery of Insulin, and the Making of a Medical Miracle by Thea Cooper and

Arthur Ainsberg. *Breakthrough* offers a new, richly detailed, and deeply personal perspective of one young girl—Elizabeth Hughes—and her family's struggle to keep her alive on a starvation diet so that she might one day enjoy a miracle: the discovery of insulin.

Cheating Destiny by James S. Hirsch. "My son is thirsty." So begins *Cheating Destiny*, Hirsch's amazing book about living with type 1 diabetes, being the parent of a child with diabetes, and so much more.

Diabetes Through the Looking Glass: Seeing Diabetes From Your Child's Perspective by Dr. Rachel Besser. Dr. Besser not only offers excellent diabetes care advice, but she also brings a unique perspective by including interviews with children and adults with type 1 diabetes.

The Discovery of Insulin by Michael Bliss. This is the definitive exploration of the work of the team in Toronto, Canada, that discovered insulin. A must read.

The Fight to Survive: A Young Girl, Diabetes, and the Discovery of Insulin by Caroline Cox. This is the personal story of Elizabeth Evans Hughes, daughter of Charles Evans Hughes, who was diagnosed with type 1 diabetes in 1919 when she was eleven years old. She was one of the first children treated with insulin.

Help with the Hard Stuff by Lauren W. Tolle, PhD, and William T. O'Donohue, PhD. This workbook for parents and teens can help make life as a teen with type 1 easier.

Kids First Diabetes Second: Tips for Parents of a Child with Type 1 Diabetes by Leighann Calentine. There are many books about the medical aspects of living with type 1. There are few about the "living a life" aspects of type 1. This is one of the best.

My Sister Has Diabetes and How That Makes Me Feel by Grace Rooney. In the twenty-six years that our family has been involved in the type 1 diabetes community, I have never encountered a resource for siblings with the depth of insight I found in this book.

Raising Teens with Diabetes: A Survival Guide for Parents by Moira McCarthy. Are you a parent of a teen with type 1 diabetes? If so, you need this book. It's as simple as that.

Think Like a Pancreas by Gary Scheiner, MS, CDE. This is one of the best manuals on day-to-day diabetes management.

101   Life Is Lived Off Label

At a Friends for Life conference in Orlando in 2012, Kendall Simmons, a former NFL offensive lineman, helped present the closing keynote address. Kendall was asked what he did if he needed insulin during a game. He said he injected through his uniform. Immediately, a representative of an insulin company stood up and noted that injecting through clothing was an off-label use of their product. Since I was serving as emcee for the closing keynote, I thanked the representative for the comment but noted, "Life is lived off label."

I mention this because it's an important part of achieving our goal of living life well with type 1 diabetes. Our goal isn't to blindly follow the approved use guidelines for a device or drug. If we did, kids under two years old wouldn't be able to use any insulin analog, insulin pump, or continuous sensor because none have been approved by the FDA for children that young. If we did, teens who struggle with weight issues wouldn't take advantage of the many newly approved drugs for adults with type 2 diabetes that allow them—under the supervision of their diabetes care team—to lose weight safely. If we did, some would have heeded the initial guidance of their care team and set aside their dreams, and the world would not know Gary Hall, Jr., as an Olympic gold medal winner, Nicole Johnson as Miss America, Charlie Kimball as an IndyCar driver, Douglas Cairns as a pilot who has flown around the world, Kendall Simmons as a Super Bowl–winning football player, and Will Cross and Sebastien Sasseville as men who have stood at the top of Mt. Everest, conquering the world.

9

The Bottom Line

Our challenge as parents is to remember that a life well-lived is the goal, and to find a way to fit diabetes into the dreams and aspirations of our children so that they may live the life of their dreams.

10

Additional Resources

10 Joanne Cunha's video: www.youtube.com/watch?v=LFIVVHQ
od5o.

Joanne's daughter was diagnosed with type 1 when she was a
baby. You can read more of Joanne's wisdom on her blog at
www.deathofapancreas.com

13 Safe Sittings: www.safesittings.com

15 ADA: www.diabetes.org; JDRF: www.jdrf.org

17 TCOYD: www.tcoyd.org; CWD: www.childrenwithdiabetes.com

20 Reputable diabetes websites: www.diabetes.org; www.jdrf.org;
www.joslin.org; www.childrenwithdiabetes.com

Understanding Diabetes: www.ucdenver.edu/academics/colleges
/medicalschool/centers/BarbaraDavis/OnlineBooks
/Pages/UnderstandingDiabetes.aspx

21 Diabetes Dad website: diabetesdad.org

27 Children with Diabetes website: www.childrenwithdiabetes
.com/d_0j_20w.htm

Hamilton Health Sciences: www.hamiltonhealthsciences.ca/ documents/Patient%20Education/GlucagonMiniDose-lw.pdf

39   ADA website: www.diabetes.org/living-with-diabetes/parents -and-kids/diabetes-care-at-school/written-care-plans/section -504-plan.html

Safe at School Program of the American Diabetes Association: www.diabetes.org/living-with-diabetes/parents-and-kids /diabetes-care-at-school/

CWD website: www.childrenwithdiabetes.com/504/

NIDDK: www.niddk.nih.gov/health-information/health -communication-programs/ndep/health-care-professionals/ school-guide/Documents/ndep61_schoolguide_bw_508.pdf

You can also download sections here: www.niddk.nih.gov /health-information/health-communication-programs/ndep /health-care-professionals/school-guide/Pages/publicationdetail .aspx#main

45   Riding on Insulin website: www.ridingoninsulin.org/contact .html

Connected in Motion website: www.connectedinmotion.ca

53   JDRF's guide on pregnancy: www.jdrf.org/wp-content/ uploads/2013 /02/Outreach_pregnancy_12-14-12.pdf

Parents and teens can learn more about drinking and diabetes at www.drinkingwithdiabetes.com

56   Diabetes Scholars Foundation: diabetesscholars.org/college -scholarship/

Team Type 1 website: teamtype1.org/gasp/

Scott and Kim Verplank Foundation: verplankfoundation.com/ scholarships/

57 ADA   website   (state   laws):   www.diabetes.org/living-with
    -diabetes/know-your-rights/discrimination/drivers-licenses/drivers
    -license-laws-by-state.html

59 You can find additional ideas at "Preparing Students With Dia-
    betes for Life at College": care.diabetesjournals.org
    /content/26/9/2675.full and "Going to College with Diabetes":
    main.diabetes.org/dorg/living-with-diabetes/edmats-lawyers
    /going-to-college-with-diabetes.pdf

60 College Diabetes Network: www.collegediabetesnetwork.org
    Students with Diabetes: studentswithdiabetes.com

69 You can read an abstract of the study online at online
    .liebertpub.com/doi/abs/10.1089/dia.2009.0112

71 Children with Diabetes: www.childrenwithdiabetes.com/clinic
    /untethered.htm

73 Nightscout: www.nightscout.info

75 You can learn more online at www.childrenwithdiabetes.com/
    ast/

76 Tartoos: myvisualmedical.com.

78 Diabetes Cure: care.diabetesjournals.org/content/20/3/244
    .abstract

84 TSA website: blog.tsa.gov/2014/04/tsa-travel-tips-travelers
    -with-diabetes.html

86 Frio Pack: www.frioinsulincoolingcase.com

91 DCCT study: www.nejm.org/doi/full/10.1056/NEJM19930
    9303291401

97 Cumberland Hospital website: cumberlandhospital.com

98 TrialNet: www.diabetestrialnet.org

100 Six Until Me: www.sixuntilme.com

Acknowledgments

Many thanks to the team at Skyhorse Publishing, first in asking me if I'd be interested in writing a book and then in helping me to do so. For someone who likes to speak and to write, writing a book proved to be more challenging than I thought.

The wisdom and guidance of a lot of very smart people are contained in these pages. My job was just to share what I have learned. While there are too many to name (and I'd likely forget someone important due to my age), I'd like to give special thanks to two people: Richard Rubin, PhD, CDE, and Betty Brackenridge, MS, RD, CDE. Richard was a pioneer in caring for the emotional side of diabetes. He and Betty authored *Sweet Kids*, the first book to show us the way to living well with type 1 diabetes. Richard and Betty showed us the way, and we are all the better as a result.

I would also like to thank everyone who has served as faculty and staff at a Friends for Life conference over the years. To a person, you represent the very best in diabetes care, and you've helped more families than you can imagine.

Everyone involved with Children with Diabetes deserves more thanks than I can ever offer. Together, we have made a profound difference.

Deep thanks go to my wife Brenda, who read the book through several times and contributed her wider and deeper wisdom. And finally to Marissa, Kathryn, and Tim, whose experiences appear within many of these tidbits.

Index

101 Tips for Parents of Kids with Diabetes

Index